SPEAK LIFE

Proverbs 18:21

Death and life are in the power of the tongue,
And those who love it will eat its fruit.

SHARON L. AMBROSE

Speak Life

www.SpeakLifeSharon.com

ISBN: 978-1-64438-686-6

All Scripture quotations, unless otherwise indicated, are taken from the Holy Bible, New King James Version., English Standard Version, New International Version, New Living Translation, New American Standard Bible

Library of Congress Cataloging in Publication Data
Ambrose, Sharon
Speak Life by Sharon Ambrose

BODY, MIND & SPIRIT / Inspiration & Personal Growth | BODY, MIND & SPIRIT / General | BODY, MIND & SPIRIT / Healing / Prayer & Spiritual
Library of Congress Control Number: 2019937216

Published by BookLocker.com, Inc., St. Petersburg, Florida, USA

Printed on acid-free paper.

BookLocker.com, Inc. 2019

First Edition

DEDICATION

With much love and affection, this book is dedicated to my children - Donovan and Imani

My grandchildren -

Sophia, ArdithRae, Xavier, Donovan Jr., Ariana and Jossalyn

CONTENTS

ACKNOWLEDGEMENTS vii

INTRODUCTION xi

FEAR 1

GLORY TO GOD 6

A SOLDIER FOR GOD 11

CHRISTMAS GIFT 17

I GIVE YOU PRAISE 22

MY FATHER.. 27

JESUS SAVES SATAN'S SLAVES..................... 31

COVENANT... 36

I LOVE YOU 41

FIGHT FOR YOUR RIGHT 47

RESTING IN GOD'S LOVE................................. 53

SPEAK LIFE-JESUS CHRIST 58

ACKNOWLEDGEMENTS

THANK YOU GOD! GLORY TO GOD!

Colossians 3:17

And whatever you do, in word or deed, do everything in the name of the Lord Jesus, giving thanks to God the Father through him.

I would like to express my very great appreciation to you, my love and best friend, Gus Barboza, for your heartfelt support, prayers, and encouragement during the writing of this project and for your exceptional work on the book covers that truly expresses your gift and your love beyond words.

Special shout out with love to Logan Barboza for the inspiration to write and work on another piece for Easter... It's in the works Logan and I will give it to you to read first. Thank you for your loving support and appreciation.

I would like to offer my special thanks to Lynne Carnivale, my friend and sister in Christ. Your captivating photography on the book cover is admirable. Thank you for your genuine and uplifting prayers, loving words, encouragement, and friendship. I'd like to give special thanks also to Brandon Carnivale, David Carnivale, Ann Barboza, and Ernest Barboza for all your loving support in word, encouragement, and prayers.

Special appreciation and love for my friend and sister in Christ, Keisha Vasquez: Thank you for all your prayers and support in life and sharing our God given gifts with one another for the cause of the Kingdom. In your words... "it's about the content"... Amen! Let God always be the content in the lives we live everyday. I look forward to sharing our God given gifts together. Claiming our Victory!

I'd like to give special thank you to all my Sisters and Brothers in Christ for their prayers and uplifting words of encouragement.

With great appreciation and love, I would like to thank my family: Carolyn Nolan my sister, one of my best friends and cheerleaders in life who lovingly supports and encourages me. Frank Nolan, Mark Ambrose, Alyssa Costa, Natalia Almeida, Shaiann Andrade and William Lewis for their prayers, loving support and encouragement in life with open hearts and minds.

Finally, to my children Donovan and Imani and grandchildren Sophia, ArdathRae, Xavier, Donovan Jr., Ariana, and Jossalyn: I am truly loved and blessed beyond measure to have each one of you as a gift from God to fill my life with love and joy and memories to carry with us forever. May we continue in our faith, running the race with endurance in life's journey together; and speaking life over each other in love and prayers. With God at the center, may we continue to carry on the legacy of our Lord and Savior Jesus Christ.

INTRODUCTION

May this heartfelt, God-inspired word fill your spirit and speak life and love into your hearts, souls, and lives. Because the enemy comes to steal, kill and destroy as stated in John 10:10, *The thief cometh not, but for to steal, and to kill, and to destroy: I am come that they might have life, and that they might have it more abundantly.*

One way he does this is by causing division in your relationships, your family, and even in your church. Luke 12:52-53 tells us this would happen: *For from now on five in one house will be divided: three against two, and two against three. The father will be divided against son and son against father, mother against daughter and daughter against mother, mother-in-law against her daughter-in-law and daughter-in-law against her mother-in-law.*

Let me ask this: What are we doing about it? Are we putting on the suit of armor every day? Are we sowing seeds into the lives of people around us or those we love? And what about our prayer life? Because I'll tell you this, the enemy really has NO power unless we give it to him. Give him nothing to work with. Claim your Victory in Jesus Christ and allow GOD to overcome the enemy. Another way we can do this is told to us right in Luke 10:19, *Behold, I give you the authority to trample on serpents and scorpions, and over all the power of the enemy, and nothing shall by any means hurt you.* That includes the devil. START STOMPING!

Moreover, because what we say or do can affect our children and relationships. Speak life over your children and your loved ones; and by doing so, bless them with love in word and in truth. 1 John 4:8 says, *He who does not love does not know God, for God is love.* In this world, I have seen hurt people who feel like the “Black Sheep” (outcast) in their own family. I am here to tell you, it’s not about being the “Black Sheep;” it’s about being “God’s Sheep” in His family. He has given us a purpose—to sow seeds for the cause of the kingdom. **Matthew 28:19, *Go therefore go and make disciples of all nations, baptizing them in the name of the Father and of the Son and of the Holy Spirit.***

1 Corinthians 13:4-8

Love is patient, love is kind. It does not envy, it does not boast, it is not proud. It does not dishonor others, it is not self-seeking, it is not easily angered, it keeps no record of wrongs. Love does not delight in evil but rejoices with the truth. It always protects, always trusts, always hopes, always perseveres.

Romans 13:8

"Owe no one anything, except to love each other, for the one who loves another has fulfilled the law."

1 Corinthians 13:13

And now abide faith, hope, love, these three; but the greatest of these is love.

FEAR

FEAR

Fear is the opposite of faith

2 Timothy says, **For God has not given us a spirit of fear, but of power and of love and of sound mind.**

Fear of emotional affliction

Fear became the addiction,

Worried about the children and family

All we have to do is pray incessantly,

The fear of life and people become an oppression

Day by day leading to an obsession

Then becoming a victim to depression

Lord, you are great with wisdom and life lessons,

Contemplated on what people would think or say

Had a hard time saying no, but it was almost every day,

This fear is approval addiction

Worried about paying bills, especially when there was no job

Worried about caring for my family;

Worry is another fear that had to stop,

Fear of relationships and friendships

Afraid to get hurt or deal with rejection

Fear is a wall that we put up for protection,

Pondered going back to college but within us is the fear of failure

All we have to do is look to you, Father, in prayer,

When we speak to you, Father, and tell you we are tired of our life, we felt stagnant;

Not because we were tired of you

Because you are our rock and refuge,

You answered our prayer, blessed us to use our gifts in ministry

You took away the fear when we had faith in you and the power to believe,

Through prayer, extended your gift of love and sent us back to college

Thank you for grace, wisdom, and knowledge

Lord, you gave us a faith we can't explain

Freed from the bondage of fears

That affected us for years,

A new life with our Savior who sets us free

Our body is your temple and you provided the Holy

Spirit within us

Father, in our storms you always see us through

Break us and mold us to be more like you,

Father, without you we are weak but with you we are strong

Through your mighty power, our fears are gone,

Fear can come in many forms

But only God almighty can get you through the storms
When your praise is high! Your worry is low!

Let God be your testimony to and fro.

Matthew 10:28

And do not fear those who kill the body but cannot kill the soul. But rather fear Him who is able to destroy both soul and body in hell.

Psalm 55:22

Cast your burden on the Lord, And He shall sustain you; He shall never permit the righteous to be moved.

Psalm 18:2

The Lord is my rock and my fortress and my deliverer; My God, my strength, in whom I will trust; My shield and the horn of my salvation, my stronghold.

Psalm 118:6

The Lord is on my side; I will not fear. What can man do to me?

GLORY TO GOD

GLORY TO GOD

Give Praise! Worthy to be praised

For all of our days!!!

My Victory in Prayer!

My Victory in Life!

My Lord and Savior!

My Lord and Savior!

Give Praise! Almighty, He is! God of the living

Father of heaven created all things,

Jehovah's Omnipotence into the heaven and earths existence

Holy! Is the God most- high, maker of my soul and being,

King of grace, his unmerited favor that pours out His kindness and love He is almighty

Lords freedom of abundant life that changes us to be free,

The first, the last, the living one

Sword of salvation,

The Great I am; highest of earthly things

He is, Alpha-Omega; the eternal nature of our being,

E'lohim! God, everlasting of the world and universe

Great High Priest and the foundation of our salvation,

Cornerstone, our shield, author and perfector of our faith

The deliverer, the great physician and bread of life that sustains,

Abba-Father! Comforter, compassion, hope and grace
Holy one of my mercy; I give Him praise!

Give Praise!

Yahweh is the revelation story

Everlasting Father, give honor and glory,

Master, the origin of the universe… blessed us with our Savior

Health of my countenance

My Victory in Prayer!

My Victory in Life!

My Lord and Savior!

My Lord and Savior!

Heavenly Father; dominion over our bodies, "His temple"

Glory in the highest! His spirit dwells in us

King of kings, fountain of living of living waters, breath of life

My fortress, my help, my judge, my Redeemer; God of true light,

Majesty is His name that heals, nourishing, provider and deliverer; Our God

Blessed hope, our guide, our potter, and letter of the law,

Yeshua! My harmony, a purpose that's significant

Heaven is beautiful because of His presence,

Lord, God infinite, righteous and pure

Holy is He that angels sing

Messiah is the freedom to share the Word! ... and shout HIS name in triumph!

Elshaddai ! Glorious God, Lord on High! Hallelujah! Give Praise! Give Praise!

My Victory in Prayer!

My Victory in Life!

My Lord and Savior!

My Victory in Prayer!

My Victory in Life!

My Lord and Savior!

My Lord and Savior!

My Victory in Prayer!

My Victory in Life!

My Lord and Savior!

My Victory in Prayer!

My Victory in Life!

My Lord and Savior!

Worthy to be praised for all of our days!

My Lord and Savior!

My Lord and Savior!

Mark 12:30

And you shall love the LORD your God with all your heart, with all your soul, with all your mind and with all your strength. This is the first commandment.

John 4:23

But the hour is coming, and now is, when the true worshipers will worship the Father in spirit and truth; for the Father is seeking such to worship Him.

Psalm 34:1

I will bless the LORD at all times: his praise shall continually be in my mouth.

1 Thessalonians 5:18

In everything give thanks; for this is the will of God in Christ Jesus for you.

Psalm 118:24

This is the day the LORD has made; We will rejoice and be glad in it.

A SOLDIER FOR GOD

A SOLDIER FOR GOD

A soldier awakes to pray

For the suit of armor to protect them in the day

The shield, the sword and helmet of salvation

That equips and empowers them to go into a worldly nation

A soldier in the storm of the valley of death will raise hands and still give praise

Gets down on his hands and knees prays

A soldier becomes all things to all men

Whether lost or a Christian

As God calls him more than a friend

He needs to proclaim the same and listen

To the commands of God!...High chieftain

A spiritual battle is every day!... once Saved!

Like a soldier!... Our Father owns us in every way.

A soldier for God is a Christian on a mission!

A soldier for God is a Christian on a mission!

A soldier for God is a Christian on a mission!

A soldier for God will help the physically and emotionally afflicted

The alcoholic, the prostitute to the drug addicted

The thief and liar from within to the physically impaired.... Shows them the Great physician

A soldier in prayer casts out demonic forces and evil divinations

Through the power of Gods inclinations

From the spiritual medium, the ouja board, the palm reader

To the tarot reader, the evil spirits and even false leaders
A soldier for God reaches out to the poor and gives to the hungry

Faith in God to provide their needs

As he walks amongst the weeds he is sowing seeds

His journey is to continue the harvest till Gods will and plan is complete

Where a murderer has given hope in repentance for his sin

Saved from a killers mind to saving lives in the pen

Becoming a fisher of men

A soldier for God is a Christian on a mission!

A soldier for God is a Christian on a mission!

A soldier for God is a Christian on a mission!

A soldier prays and loves on those considering divorce
So the faith, love and power of God will change their course

Reaches out in compassion to the abused

To give Gods hope, healing and truth

Helps the widows and orphans

Gives biblical counsel to stop abortions

Doing what God commanded him

He is not a hypocrite or a phony

He is a disciple! ... A living testimony!

When their sisters or brothers are down

Doesn't stand and gossip amongst the crowd

Doesn't throw stones in the church home

But picks them up in spiritual unconditional love and pray

To help carry them in their faith

A soldier for God will share the love of Christ and forgive his enemies

Remembering Jesus died on Calvary to set us free

He will love on purpose

Because that is the love of Jesus

A soldier for God is a Christian on a mission!

A soldier for God is a Christian on a mission!

A soldier for God is a Christian on a mission!

A soldiers' ambition

Is the Great Commission

Go make disciples!... Fear is not a decision

Lives out of the box and goes where God wants him to go

Because he doesn't know

What the future holds for tomorrow…

As Soldiers!... Are we on the fence lukewarm?

Or are we standing on the Rock in the storm?

Are we fighting the Good fight!?

So we can be Salt in the Light!

Harvesting with Christ!

Are we the bystander on the sidelines wasting time? ...

Are we with God on the front lines planting seeds in the weeds

To put branches on the vine,

A soldier for God is a Christian on a mission!

A soldier for God is a Christian on a mission!

A Christian on a mission!

A Christian on a mission!

A Christian on a mission!

Matthew 5:16

Let your light so shine before men, that they may see your good works and glorify your Father in heaven.

Matthew 28:19-20

Go therefore and make disciples of all the nations, baptizing them in the name of the Father, and of the Son, and of the Holy Spirit. Teaching them to observe all the things I have commanded you; and lo, I am with you always, even to the end of the age.

Proverbs 11:30

The fruit of the righteous is a tree of life, And he who wins souls is wise.

CHRISTMAS GIFT

CHRISTMAS GIFT

Christmas! … A celebration of our Lord Saviors birth

Red ... Color of Christmas that covers holiday on earth,

Presents are bought and wrapped with a bow and nestled under the tree

Ultimate gift from heaven; our Salvation given free

Red; the color that covers the bloodshed of our King,

Our Lord paid the price

Paid it all; His life as sacrifice,

Jesus! The way, the truth and the light of heavenly realms that glow

He washed our sins away; cleansed us white as snow,

Jesus Christ is the Christmas Story! ..Give Glory! Glory!

Jesus Christ is the Christmas Story! ..Give Glory! Glory!

Jesus Christ is the Christmas Story! ..Give Glory! Glory!

We are saved! Angels are partying in the heavens above

Oh! The melody, the joy, the peace and love

Harmonious sounds and flying doves,

Hear the Angels singing

Church bells ringing,

Harps are playing by joyful faces

Clapping, dancing and giving praises,

Trumpets are boldly sounding

Hear the drummers pounding,

Chimes are tingling a melodious tune

All for Christ love for you,

Christmas Gift! A Heavenly Home

Meeting Christ the King at His Heavenly Throne,

Celebrate our Lord every day

Share Christ with everyone; So all may be saved…
Christ is the Christmas story! Praise God! Glory! Glory!

Christ is the Christmas story!

Praise God! Glory! Glory!

Praise God! Glory! Glory!

Praise God! Glory! Glory!

Matthew 1: 18- 25

[18]Now the birth of Jesus Christ was as follows: After His
mother Mary was betrothed to Joseph, before they came
together, she was found with child of the Holy Spirit.
[19]Then Joseph her husband, being a just man, and not
wanting to make her a public example, was minded to
put her away secretly. [20]But while he thought about these
things, behold, an angel of the Lord appeared to him in
a dream, saying, "Joseph, son of David, do not be afraid
to take to you Mary your wife, for that which is
conceived in her is of the Holy Spirit. [21]And she will
bring forth a Son, and you shall call His name JESUS,
for He will save His people from their sins."[22]So all this
was done that it might be fulfilled which was spoken by
the Lord through the prophet, saying: [23]"Behold, the
virgin shall be with child, and bear a Son, and they shall
call His name Immanuel," which is translated, "God
with us." Then Joseph, being aroused from sleep, did as
the angel of the Lord commanded him and took to him
his wife, [25]and did not know her till she had brought
forth her firstborn Son. And he called His name JESUS.

Matthew 2:1-12

[1]Now after Jesus was born in Bethlehem of Judea in the
days of Herod the king, behold, wise men from the East
came to Jerusalem, saying, [2]"Where is He who has been
born King of the Jews? For we have seen His star in the
East and have come to worship Him." [3]When Herod the
king heard this, he was troubled, and all Jerusalem with
him. [4]And when he had gathered all the chief priests and
scribes of the people together, he inquired of them where
the Christ was to be born. [5]So they said to him, "In
Bethlehem of Judea, for thus it is written by the prophet:

*[6]But you, Bethlehem, in the land of Judah, Are not the
least among the rulers of Judah; For out of you shall
come a Ruler Who will shepherd My people Israel.'"
[7]Then Herod, when he had secretly called the wise men,
determined from them what time the star appeared. [8]And
he sent them to Bethlehem and said, "Go and search
carefully for the young Child, and when you have found
Him, bring back word to me, that I may come and
worship Him also." [9]When they heard the king, they
departed; and behold, the star which they had seen in
the East went before them, till it came and stood over
where the young Child was. [10]When they saw the star,
they rejoiced with exceedingly great joy. [11]And when
they had come into the house, they saw the young Child
with Mary His mother, and fell down and worshiped
Him. And when they had opened their treasures, they
presented gifts to Him: gold, frankincense, and myrrh.
[12]Then, being divinely warned in a dream that they
should not return to Herod, they departed for their own
country another way.*

I GIVE YOU PRAISE

I GIVE YOU PRAISE

Lord, you've taken me places I never dreamed of

Given me endless grace and love,

Your powerful guidance that shows me the way

I give you Praise!

Living free in your presence… eternally

Given me the truth from the book of life

My secure covenant I'm married to you beyond the earthly wife,

Searching for a stronger faith; not settling for a faith of a mustard seed

You take all my burdens and keep me from amongst the weeds,

I'm yearning for you more each day

As I am blessed to speak with you and pray

I give you Praise!

I can talk with you when the night has come You're there to console me through the comfort of your son,

The day comes and goes and I'm at rest

Because I have a Father who loves me and knows what's best,

Each new day you put a smile on my face

Because I have you by my side as I run the race…

I give you Praise!

Father you continually fill me with the Holy Spirit
within my soul

So my heart does not become cold,

Forgiveness for my weakness

Given me hope in prayer so I don't give in to fleshly sin,

You continue the spiritual battle with me so I can live
with you in Heaven…

I give you Praise!

I give you Praise!

I give you Praise!

Revelation 4:11

"You are worthy, O Lord,
To receive glory and honor and power;
For You created all things,
And by Your will they exist and were created."

Psalm 95:1-3

Oh come, let us sing to the LORD!
Let us shout joyfully to the Rock of our salvation.
Let us come before His presence with thanksgiving;
Let us shout joyfully to Him with psalms.
For the LORD is the great God,
And the great King above all gods.

Psalm 150:1-2

Praise the LORD!
Praise God in His sanctuary;
Praise Him in His mighty firmament!
Praise Him for His mighty acts; Praise Him according to His excellent greatness!

1 Thessalonians 5:18-23

In everything give thanks; for this is the will of God in Christ Jesus for you.
Do not quench the Spirit. Do not despise prophecies.
Test all things; hold fast what is good. Abstain from every form of evil.
Now may the God of peace Himself sanctify you completely; and may your whole spirit, soul, and

body be preserved blameless at the coming of our Lord Jesus Christ.

Psalm 148

Praise the LORD!
Praise the LORD from the heavens; Praise Him in the heights!
Praise Him, all His angels; Praise Him, all His hosts!
Praise Him, sun and moon;
Praise Him, all you stars of light! Praise Him, you heavens of heavens, And you waters above the heavens!
Let them praise the name of the LORD, For He commanded, and they were created.
He also established them forever and ever
He made a decree which shall not pass away.
Praise the LORD from the earth,
You great sea creatures and all the depths;
Fire and hail, snow and clouds;
Stormy wind, fulfilling His word;
Mountains and all hills;
Fruitful trees and all cedars;
Beasts and all cattle;
Creeping things and flying fowl;
Kings of the earth and all peoples;
Princes and all judges of the earth; Both young men and maidens; Old men and children.
Let them praise the name of the LORD, For His name alone is exalted;
His glory is above the earth and heaven.
And He has exalted the horn of His people,
The praise of all His saints— Of the children of Israel, A people near to Him.
Praise the LORD!

MY FATHER

MY FATHER

I am who my Father says I am

I am a child of a King

I am a parent who is passing down my Father's legacy

To the children in my family,

I am the child, my Father is molding

With His loving guidance and spiritual scolding,

I am a Christian desiring for their family to be saved

I am the child of God, who needs their Father to lead the way,

I am a Christian who prays for others

But all Christians need prayers from their sisters and brothers,

I am the Christian in the Spirit, He created me to be

As a child in the flesh He continually sets me free,

I am the child, my Father forgives

As I continue to live,

I am sinner walking in the Spirit and the flesh

Jesus Christ my Redeemer makes me clean with his

Holiness,

Saved, Baptized and renewed in the

Father, Son and Holy Spirit in water

We are the Father's sons and daughters....

Ecclesiastes 3:11

He has made everything beautiful in its time.

Romans 8:1-11

There is therefore now no condemnation to those who are in Christ Jesus, who do not walk according to the flesh, but according to the Spirit. For the law of the Spirit of life in Christ Jesus has made me free from the law of sin and death. For what the law could not do in that it was weak through the flesh, God did by sending His own Son in the likeness of sinful flesh, on account of sin: He condemned sin in the flesh, that the righteous requirement of the law might be fulfilled in us who do not walk according to the flesh but according to the Spirit. For those who live according to the flesh set their minds on the things of the flesh, but those who live according to the Spirit, the things of the Spirit. For to be carnally minded is death, but to be spiritually minded is life and peace. Because the carnal mind is enmity against God; for it is not subject to the law of God, nor indeed can be. So then, those who are in the flesh cannot please God.

But you are not in the flesh but in the Spirit, if indeed the Spirit of God dwells in you. Now if anyone does not have the Spirit of Christ, he is not His. And if Christ is in you, the body is dead because of sin, but the Spirit is life because of righteousness. But if the Spirit of Him who raised Jesus from the dead dwells in you, He who raised Christ from the dead will also give life to your mortal bodies through His Spirit who dwells in you.

Jeremiah 29:11

For I know the thoughts that I think toward you, says the LORD, thoughts of peace and not of evil, to give you a future and a hope.

Proverbs 16:9

A man's heart plans his way, But the LORD directs his steps.

Matthew 18:18-20

"Truly I tell you, whatever you bind on earth will be bound in heaven, and whatever you loose on earth will be loosed in heaven. "Again, truly I tell you that if two of you on earth agree about anything they ask for, it will be done for them by my Father in heaven. For where two or three gather in my name, there am I with them."

JESUS SAVES SATAN'S SLAVES

JESUS SAVES SATAN'S SLAVES

One day calling out to God, my Father

Sighing in the darkness

Asking for forgiveness,

Crying as times goes by

Someone is there to show me the truth from the Bible and comparing verses

From prayers to visiting Churches,

Then I was saved and saved from a false religion

Who changes the Word of the Good Book! What a sin!

They even changed the eighteenth and nineteenth

Revelation warning verse

Father didn't they know this is a deadly curse,

It says," **If anyone adds to these things, God will add to him the plagues that are written in this book.**

And if anyone takes away from the words of the book of this prophecy, God shall take away his part in the Book of Life.

Thank you! … Lord for blessing me and saving my life.

Once saved, the battle started with the devil from day one

Words from a cult rolling off their lips

Then I had to realize I'm a child of God, not their little kid,

It wasn't about who was right or wrong

It was about the book of John,

Verse 3:16 (NKJV) For God so loved the world that He gave His only begotten Son. That whoever believes in him should not perish, but have everlasting life.

They were mad about the scriptures I read

Had no idea they were being spiritually fed,
No longer a part of my life

Now I'm praying for Christ to give them life,

During time was taken from the bondage of clubs

Realizing nothing was really there

Because it was like being in the devils house where no one really cares

Thank you Lord for being there,

Instead I can look forward to Gods' house in heaven

More trials to come, satan doesn't sleep- neither does

God… twenty- four seven,

Tried to move to have a better life;
received nothing but headaches and people causing strife,

Bitterness from people who couldn't see me free

Thank you God for the suit of armor that shields me in reality,

Ephesians 6:11 Put on the whole armor of God that you may be able to stand against the wiles of the devil.

In my walk with you Father, I battled with depression

Along the way you showed me a life lesson,

Not to just think of myself

To get up and help someone else,

Because the whole world is not yet saved

You put your sheep here for a purpose … just show us the way,

I'm not perfect like your heavenly angels

Yet you forgave me, loved me and saved me…

If you don't have Christ

In your life,

I hope you accept him in prayer

To be saved and blessed by our Lord and Savior!

We all have a testimonial story

But in the end … God gets the Glory!

John 3:16

For God so loved the world that He gave his only begotten son, that whoever believes in Him, should not perish, but have everlasting life.

John 14:6

Jesus said to him, "I am the way, the truth, and the life. No one comes to the Father except through Me."

John 10:28-30

"And I give them eternal life, and they shall never perish; neither shall anyone snatch them out of My hand. My Father, who has given them to me, is greater than all; and no one is able to snatch them out of My Father's hand. I and My Father are one."

SALVATION PRAYER

Father, in the name of Jesus, I ask You to forgive all my sins. Jesus, come into my heart and live in me. Thank You, Jesus, for coming into my heart. Thank You that all my sins are forgiven and that I have been born again.

Amen!

COVENANT

COVENANT

A covenant for us, through Jesus precious blood

A living sacrifice for the sins of the world
A permanent binding relationship with God and Jesus the son,

A covenant eternally- The Holy one,

We are blessed because we're the object of His love and grace

Lord, your word tells us we are valuable

Precious in your sight,

At times we don't feel worthy and yet given us

Prayer of forgiveness to make us right,

Forgave us and molded us to walk in your image

Chosen to receive your love and blessings

Made Holy when you forgave us for our sins,

God calls us more than a friend

We're named in His will to receive a royal inheritance,

Marked with a seal

Of the Holy Spirit that's so real,

A covenant hope that knows God is faithful

Will not leave you or forsake you,

Keeps His covenant unlike any human on earth

The Lord will never let you down

We're showered with His beauty and love so proud,

God has called your name

Calling you to live in heavenly places on a higher plane

When your heart is open to that calling

You'll never be the same,

A covenant where our sins and "lawless deeds"

Are remembered no more

A robe of purity is put on that only He adores,

Sprinkled our hearts clean from a guilty conscience

Believer! Jesus Christ has wrapped you in a robe
A garment of His salvation

A robe of righteousness from a heavenly nation,

Like Joseph, you wear the coat of a blessed child

Like Tamar, you wear the long sleeved garment of the virgin daughter of the King

Who awaits purely for her wedding ring,

Like the Kings of Israel and Judah you are arrayed

In royal robes and seated with Christ in heavenly places

A covenant not exchanged but given upon graces,

Like Esther, you are wearing royal robes since you are the bride of the King of kings

The Father makes you into a Holy Queen,

Like the Prodigal son; God your Father has forgiven you, exchanged your filthy rags for a family robe;

Forgiven, redeemed and restored

Now we are secure,

Lord Jesus, thank you for clothing me

In garments of Salvation and wrapping me in your identity,

An oath of solemn promise when we confess

Our acceptance,

Jesus as Lord

You enter into a covenant with God as He enters into a

Covenant with you…

Matthew 10:32

"Therefore whoever confesses me before men, him I will also confess before my Father who is in heaven."

Isaiah 59:21

As for me, this is my covenant with them, saith the LORD; my spirit that is upon thee, and my words which I have put in thy mouth, shall not depart out of thy mouth, nor out of the mouth of thy seed, nor out of the mouth of thy seed's seed, saith the LORD, from henceforth and forever.

Isaiah 40:8

The grass withereth, the flower fadeth: but the word of our God shall stand for ever.

SALVATION PRAYER

Father, in the name of Jesus, I ask You to forgive all my sins. Jesus, come into my heart and live in me. Thank You, Jesus, for coming into my heart. Thank You that all my sins are forgiven and that I have been born again.

Amen!

I LOVE YOU

I LOVE YOU

To love you

To love you the way GOD intended me to,

To be the blessed gift of love

A love you could never experience, but through GOD above,

The gift of a love blessing is bestowed upon you

The desires of your heart that only GOD can fulfill

To love you according to his word, purpose, plan and will,

To love you is to abide in GOD, to edify you, encourage you

Uplift you, enhance you as GOD has called me to do,

To be a compliment to you and your life

To love you as the added blessing I am divinely called to be

Living through our Victory,

To love you is proclaiming to live GODS love right

To love you is making GOD the center and stronghold of our hearts and life,

To love you, is being a good steward over our relationship with GOD, in word and in prayer
To love you as GOD approves,

To love you is being evenly yoked

We can share the same GOD given love he provides

Love with GOD is one that is endless and never subsides,

To become a love that grows spiritually with you

To love you as GOD created me to

When we become one

GODS' will and plan is done….

WANT GODS LOVE TO BE AT WORK IN YOUR RELATIONSHIPS!

REFLECT GODS' LOVE!

GLORIFY GOD WITH YOUR RELATIONSHIPS!

1 Corinthians 13:4-8

Love is patient, love is kind. It does not envy, it does not boast, it is not proud. It does not dishonor others, it is not self-seeking, it is not easily angered, it keeps no record of wrongs. Love does not delight in evil but rejoices with the truth. It always protects, always trusts, always hopes, always perseveres. Love never fails. But where there are prophecies, they will cease; where there are tongues, they will be stilled; where there is knowledge, it will pass away.

1 Corinthians 13:13

And now abide faith, hope, love, these three; but the greatest of these is love.

Romans 13:8

"Owe no one anything, except to love each other, for the one who loves another has fulfilled the law."

Genesis 2:24

Therefore a man shall leave his father and mother and be joined to his wife, and they shall become one flesh.

Ephesians 5:22-33

Wives, submit to your own husbands, as to the Lord. For the husband is head of the wife, as also Christ is head of the church; and He is the Savior of the body. Therefore, just as the church is subject to Christ, so let the wives be to their own husbands in everything.

Husbands, love your wives, just as Christ also loved the church and gave Himself for her, that He might sanctify and cleanse her with the washing of water by the word, that He might present her to Himself a glorious church, not having spot or wrinkle or any such thing, but that she should be holy and without blemish. So husbands ought to love their own wives as their own bodies; he who loves his wife loves himself. For no one ever hated his own flesh, but nourishes and cherishes it, just as the Lord does the church. For we are members of His body, of His flesh and of His bones. "For this reason a man shall leave his father and mother and be joined to his wife, and the two shall become one flesh." This is a great mystery, but I speak concerning Christ and the church. Nevertheless let each one of you in particular so love his own wife as himself, and let the wife see that she respects her husband.

Psalm 112:1-2

Blessed is the man who fears the Lord, Who delights greatly in His commandments. His descendants will be mighty on earth;
The generation of the upright will be blessed Praise the Lord.

Proverbs 18:22

He who finds a wife finds a good thing, And obtains favor from the LORD.

Malachi 2:15

But did He not make them one, Having a remnant of the Spirit? And why one?
He seeks godly offspring.
Therefore take heed to your spirit, And let none deal treacherously with the wife of his youth.

Genesis 1:28

Then God blessed them, and God said to them, "Be fruitful and multiply; fill the earth and subdue it; have dominion over the fish of the sea, over the birds of the air, and over every living thing that moves on the earth."

1 Peter 3:7

Husbands, likewise, dwell with them with understanding, giving honor to the wife, as to the
weaker vessel, and as being heirs together of the grace of life, that your prayers may not be hindered.

2 Corinthians 6:14

Do not be unequally yoked together with unbelievers.
For what fellowship has righteousness with lawlessness?
And what communion has light with darkness?

Mark 10:9

"Therefore what God has joined together, let not man separate."

FIGHT FOR YOUR RIGHT

FIGHT FOR YOUR RIGHT

The enemy comes in disguise

Filling your head with lies,

Anger, fear, un-forgiveness, hurt and depression is an illusion

The enemy uses to cause confusion,

Making the wrong decisions

Ending up in prison,

Thinking there's nothing to live for

Looking to go hard core,

Joining a gang or a becoming a thug

Getting high or selling drugs

Drinking and visiting clubs,

Suicide- Murder- Guns

Stealing just for fun,

The battle field is in the mind where the war begins

It's up to you whether or not you commit the sin,

God! …will help you check yourself
Before you wreck yourself!

Fight for your right

To be like Christ

Because it's your life!

The truth in reality is you're Gods' sheep

To be a living testimony

To carry on Jesus legacy

Upon your family tree,

Giving you a life

To live for Christ,

The Victory

That sets all free….

John 8:36 If the son therefore shall make you free; you shall be free indeed. (NKJV)

Fight for your right

To be like Christ

Because it's your life!

The truth in reality is you're Gods' sheep

To be a living testimony

To carry on Jesus legacy

Upon your family tree,

Giving you a life

To live for Christ,

The Victory

That sets all free….

Have you been waiting for a blessing? ...A miracle?

God is your greatest blessing and miracle!

Have you been looking for direction? … Or an answer?
God is the answer!
Have you been looking for a sign?
God is giving you one today!
You are not here by accident
God has a purpose for your life!
Fight for your right
To be like Christ
Because it's your life!

Romans 12:2

Do not be conformed to this world, but be transformed by the renewing of your mind, that you may prove what is that good and acceptable and perfect will of God.

Jeremiah 29:11

For I know the thoughts that I think toward you, says the LORD, thoughts of peace and not of evil, to give you a future and a hope.

Ephesians 6:12

For we do not wrestle against flesh and blood, but against principalities, against powers, against the rulers of the darkness of this age, against spiritual hosts of wickedness in the heavenly places.

Luke 10:19

Behold, I give you the authority to trample on serpents and scorpions, and over all the power of the enemy, and nothing shall by any means hurt you.

1 Corinthians 15:57

But thanks be to God, who gives us the victory through our Lord Jesus Christ.

John 3:16

For God so loved the world that He gave his only begotten son, that whoever believes in Him, should not perish, but have everlasting life.

SALVATION PRAYER

Father, in the name of Jesus, I ask You to forgive all my sins. Jesus, come into my heart and live in me. Thank You, Jesus, for coming into my heart. Thank You that all my sins are forgiven and that I have been born again.

Amen!

"Fight For Your Right" was written in 2017 for the young men who are residents at the Taunton Detention Center (Goss Building) Taunton, Ma.

RESTING IN GOD'S LOVE

RESTING IN GOD'S LOVE

Father you embrace me with your arms
Shield me and protect me from worldly charms,
When I'm down you lift me up
Holding on to you, you're enough
Resting in Gods' love,
You bring a smile to my face
Joyful singing and giving you praise,
When trials are all upside down
You keep my feet up from the ground,
You hold on to my hand when I had enough
Resting in Gods' love!
You give me hope! Give me faith! Give me love!
You give me a song to sing!
God! You're all I need!
Your wisdom! Your power! Your almighty!
You're glorious! You're glorious!
Waiting to see my Savior in the heavens above
Resting in Gods' love....
You're enough... you're enough..
You're enough for me....
Resting in Gods' love!
God is enough!

Christ died on Calvary
Given his life for me
Lord rescued me!... Saved me!...
Now I'm free!...
Loving you! Loving you! Eternally!
Resting in Gods' love
You're enough… you're enough,,,
You're enough for me
Lord you're the one I adore
Yet, you always love me more,
You seek me out when I am lost
It's the Holy power of the Cross,
Father, you meet me when I pray
You are talking to me every day,
You give me hope! Give me faith! Give me love!
You give me a song to sing!
God! You're all I need!
Your wisdom! Your power! Your almighty!
You're glorious! You're glorious!
Waiting to see my Savior in the heavens above
Resting in Gods' love….
You're enough… you're enough..
You're enough for me….
Resting in Gods' love!
God is enough!

Psalm 23

*The LORD is my shepherd; I shall not want.
He makes me to lie down in green pastures; He leads me beside the still waters. He restores my soul;
He leads me in the paths of righteousness For His name's sake. Yea, though I walk through the valley of the shadow of death, I will fear no evil; For You are with me; Your rod and Your staff, they comfort me.
You prepare a table before me in the presence of my enemies; You anoint my head with oil; My cup runs over. Surely goodness and mercy shall follow me all the days of my life; And I will dwell in the house of the LORD Forever.*

Psalms 91:1

He who dwells in the secret place of the Most High shall abide under the shadow of the Almighty.

Matthew 11:28

Come to Me, all you who labor and are heavy laden, and I will give you rest.

Proverbs 3:5-6

*Trust in the LORD with all your heart,
And lean not on your own understanding; In all your ways acknowledge Him, And He shall direct your paths.*

Psalm 55:22

Cast your burden on the Lord, And He shall sustain you; He shall never permit the righteous to be moved.

Isaiah 55:11

So shall My word be that goes forth from My mouth; It shall not return to Me void, But it shall accomplish what I please, And it shall prosper in the thing for which I sent it.

1 John 4:9-10

In this the love of God was manifested toward us, that God has sent His only begotten Son into the world, that we might live through Him. In this is love, not that we loved God, but that He loved us and sent His Son to be the propitiation for our sins.

SPEAK LIFE-JESUS CHRIST

SPEAK LIFE-JESUS CHRIST

Death and life are in the power of the tongue,

And those who love it will eat its fruit.

Let your speech always be with grace, as though seasoned with salt, so that you will know how you should respond to each person

It is better to dwell in the wilderness, than with a contentious and an angry woman,

For we all stumble in many things. And if anyone does not stumble in word, he is a perfect man, able also to bridle the whole body

The tongue of the wise commends knowledge, but the mouths of fools pours out folly,

Gracious words are like a honeycomb, sweetness to the soul and health to the body,

For God gave us a spirit not of fear, but of power and love and self-control

A fool's mouth is his ruin, and his lips are a snare to his soul,

For whoever desires to love life and see good days, let him keep his tongue from evil and his lips from speaking deceit;

I tell you, on the day of judgement people will give account for every careless word they speak...

SPEAK LIFE-JESUS CHRIST

Let no corrupting talk come out of your mouths
but only such as is good
for building up as fits the occasion

It may give grace to those who listen,

The words of a wise man's mouth win him favor, but the lips of a fool consume him

Whoever restrains his words has knowledge, and he who has a cool spirit is a man of understanding.

Let there be no filthiness nor foolish talk nor crude joking, which are out of place, but instead let there be thanksgiving.

Do you see a man who is hasty in his words? There is more hope for a fool than for him

Whoever guards his mouth preserves his life; he who opens wide his lips comes to ruin

Know this, my beloved brothers: let every person be quick to hear, slow to speak, slow to anger for

The LORD will keep you from all DANGER-- he will watch over your life

A soft answer turns away wrath, but a harsh word stirs up anger

Do not speak evil against one another, brothers. The one who speaks against a brother or judges his brother,

speaks evil against the law and judges the law. But if you judge the law, you are not a doer of the law but a judge

Do not seek revenge or bear a GRUDGE against anyone among your people, but love your neighbor as yourself. I am the LORD.

Fulfil ye my joy, that ye be like-minded, having the same love, being of one ACCORD, of one mind.

Hypocrite! First cast out the beam from your eye, and then you will see clearly to cast out the splinter from the eye of your brother

Therefore, having put away falsehood, let each one of you speak the truth with his neighbor, for we are members one of another,

They were filled with all manner of unrighteousness, evil, covetousness, malice. They are full of envy, murder, strife, deceit, maliciousness. They are gossips

Their throat is an open grave; they use their tongues to deceive. The venom of asps is under their lips.

A gentle tongue is a tree of life, but perverseness in it breaks the spirit,

And they were all filled with the Holy Spirit and began to speak in other tongues as the Spirit gave them utterance.

For by your words you will be justified, and by your words you will be condemned.

The words of the wicked are to lie in wait for blood: but the mouth of the upright shall deliver them

The mouth of the righteous is a fountain of life, but the mouth of the wicked conceals violence

Do not merely listen to the word, and so deceive yourselves. Do what it says.

Do not repay evil for evil or reviling for reviling, but on the contrary, bless,

for to this you were called, that you may obtain a blessing

Who is wise and understanding among you?

By his good conduct let him show his works in the meekness of wisdom,

And the tongue is a fire, a world of iniquity: so is the tongue among our members, that it defileth the whole body, and setteth on fire the course of nature; and it is set on fire of hell

Only let your manner of life be worthy of the gospel of

Christ, so that whether I come and see you or am absent, I may hear of you that you are standing firm in one spirit, with one mind striving side by side for The faith of the gospel,

A wise man will hear, and will increase learning; and a man of understanding shall attain unto wise counsel,

The good person out of the good treasure of his heart produces good, and the evil person out of his evil

treasure produces evil, for out of the abundance of the

heart his mouth speaks

SPEAK LIFE-JESUS CHRIST

But I say to you that everyone who is angry with his brother will be liable to judgment; whoever insults his brother will be liable to the council; and whoever says, 'You fool!' will be liable to the hell of fire

Human anger does not produce the righteousness God desires

So also the tongue is a small member, yet it boasts of great things. How great a forest is set ablaze by such a small fire,

Whoever spares the rod hates his son, but he who loves him is diligent to discipline him

In your anger do not sin,

Therefore he who is prudent will keep silent in such a time, for it is an evil…time

For this is the will of God, that by doing good you may put to silence the ignorance of foolish men

As for the scoundrel—his devices are evil; he plans wicked schemes to ruin the poor with lying words, even when the plea of the needy is right

It is the Spirit who gives life; the flesh profits nothing. The words that I speak to you are spirit, and they are life.

SPEAK LIFE-JESUS CHRIST

Fathers, do not provoke your children, lest they become discouraged

But this again did even forget his own strength, that the righteous might be nourished,

Do your best to present yourself to God as one approved, a worker who has no need to be ashamed, rightly handling the word of truth,

So put away all malice and all deceit and hypocrisy and envy and all slander.

Better is a poor man who walks in his integrity . Than he who is perverse in speech and is a fool

God is a Spirit: and they that worship him must worship him in spirit and in truth

Every good and perfect gift is from above, coming down from the Father of the heavenly lights, who does not change like shifting shadows

Do not be deceived: God cannot be mocked.

A man reaps what he sows,

But thanks be to God, who gives us the victory through our Lord Jesus Christ!

SPEAK LIFE-JESUS CHRIST

Hebrews 13:8

Jesus Christ is the same yesterday, today, and forever. (NKJV)

Isaiah 40:8

"The grass withers, the flower fades, But the word of our God stands forever." (NKJV)

CPSIA information can be obtained
at www.ICGtesting.com
Printed in the USA
FFHW021104080619
52857977-58441FF

9 781644 386866